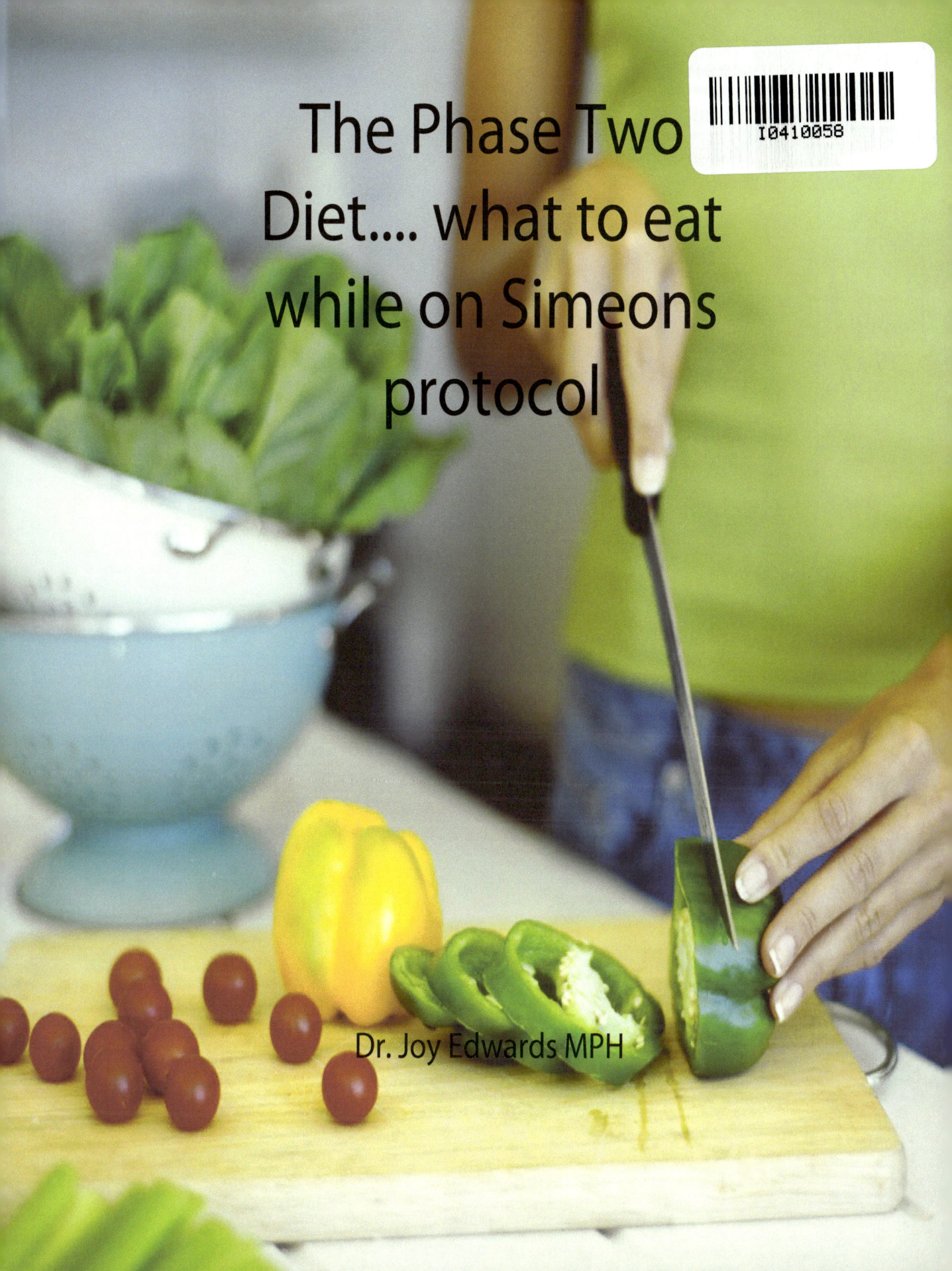

# The Phase Two Diet.... what to eat while on Simeons protocol

Dr. Joy Edwards MPH

# DEDICATION

To my beautiful angel AYANNA. Without your birth and death my
journey to wellness would have never have begun

Love always your mommy

# CONTENTS

# ACKNOWLEDGMENTS

Thank you to Dr. Simeons protocol
Thank you to Satori Tufts for her editing skills

# Chapter One

## Seafood dishes

As you know with the choices of Shrimp/Lobster Crab or White fish this tends to be the yummiest of the three when it comes to food ideas.

Remember, any fish that is white is allowed.
No canned fish, no salmon, pickled or fried fish is allowed during phase two.

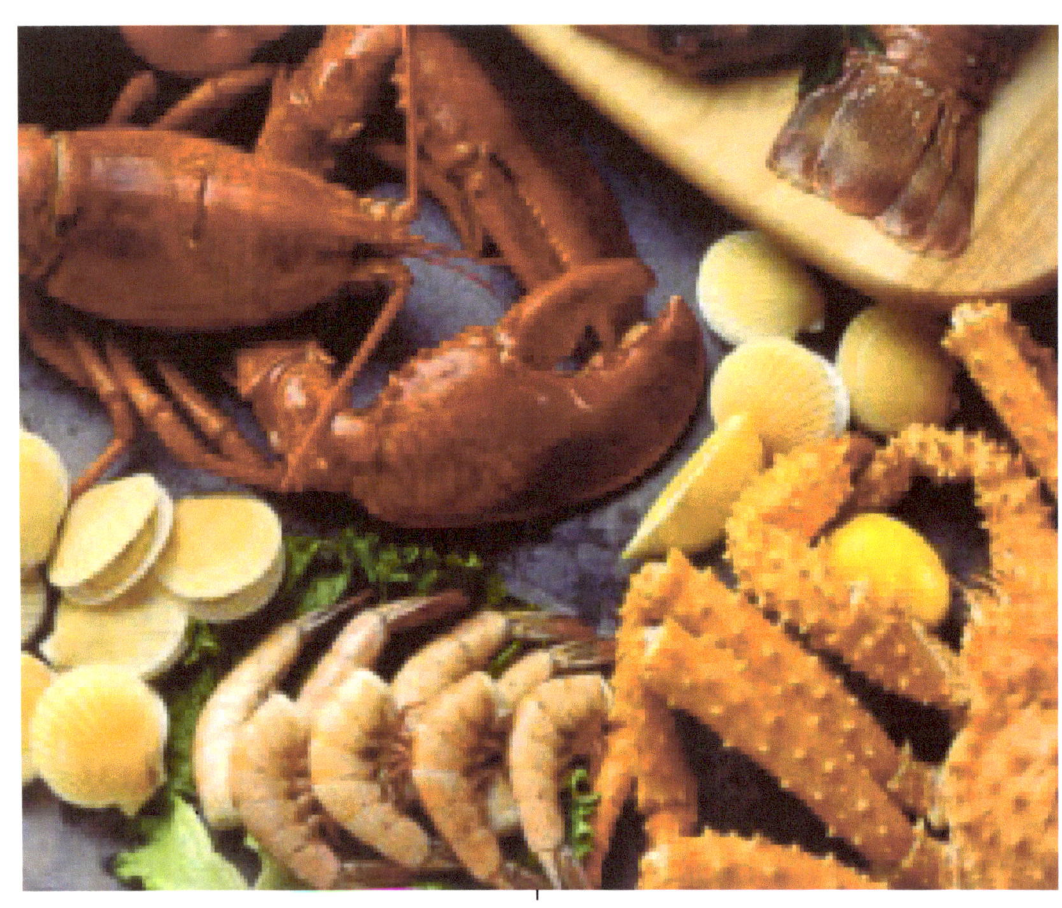

# Baked Lobster with Pesto Recipe

This baked lobster recipe is incredibly simple and delicious. The basic recipe also works well with crabmeat or other seafood.

## Ingredients

100 g cooked lobster meat (boiled, baked or grilled)
serving of any of veggies on phase two allowed list
1 tbsp of garlic powder, basil
1/2 cup chicken stock (free range organic) or fresh broth from lobsters
salt and red pepper to taste

## Instructions

In a medium casserole dish, Add lobster meat and stir.
Coat with garlic powder broth and basil mix, adding extra if desired. Put in oven at 350 degrees for 15 minutes.

# HCG DIET RECIPE BOOK

# Tasty Sea Bass

Ingredients:

- 100g of sea bass fillets
- 2 cloves garlic, minced
- 1/2 of lemon
- 1/2 tsp. salt
- 1/2 tsp. lemon pepper
- 2 tbsp finely chopped cilantro
- 1/2 tsp. paprika

Directions:

- Arrange sea bass fillets in a single layer on foil-lined broiler pan. Spread garlic and cilantro on and around fish. Squeeze lemon juice on fillets, sprinkle salt and lemon pepper to taste, and add paprika for color. Cover with foil and crimp edges to form a seal. Bake at 450 for 20 minutes.

# Seafood Chowder

Ingredients:

- 1 (14.5 ounce) can diced tomatoes
- 3 stalks celery, chopped
- 1 teaspoon dried oregano
- 1 teaspoon dried basil
- Salt and pepper to taste
- 100g of frozen cod fillets you can also put lobster or crab or shrimp in place of the cod
- This is enough to save and eat for a meal the next day

Directions:

- In a medium sized pot place un-drained tomatoes, celery, oregano, basil, salt and pepper. Bring to a boil over medium heat. Place seafood (one type) in pot. Reduce heat and cook for 10 to 15 minutes. Cook until mixture is heated through and fish is opaque and flaky. Thin with a little water if desired.

# Seafood Stuffed Tomato

- 100g cooked shrimp (can be substituted with white fish, Lobster or crab)
- Tomato – allowed amount (one large)
- Juice of half lemon
- 1 tbsp parsley (and any additional seasonings you like)
- Salt/pepper to taste
- Hot sauce (optional)

Chop up shrimp. Or, simply chop with sharp knife. In small bowl, combine chopped shrimp, parsley, lemon juice, and salt/pepper. Cover and refrigerate 30 mins-1 hr. When ready to serve, cut off top of tomato. Scoop out inside of tomato. Chop & combine inside of tomato with shrimp mix. Fill tomato with shrimp mix. Top with a couple dashes of Tabasco (optional) and serve.

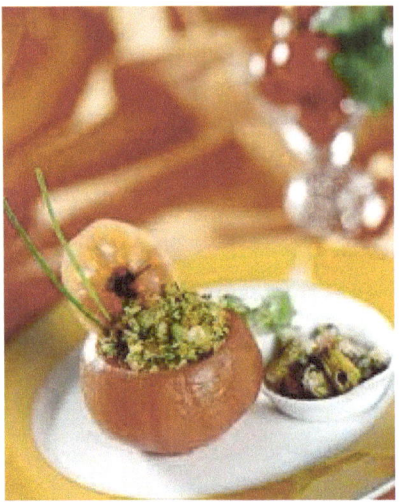

# Tangy Crab Cucumber Salad

- 100g crab – shredded
- Cucumber – peeled, seeded, (1 medium)
- 1/2 tbsp rice vinegar
- 1/2-1 tbsp spicy mustard
- 1/2-1 tsp wasabi powder
- 1 Grissini/or 1melba toast – coarsely ground

Combine rice vinegar, spicy mustard, and wasabi powder. Stir.
Add remaining ingredients, toss & serve.


includes your meat, veggie, and Melba toast portion for this meal

# Curry Shrimp

- 100g shrimp
- Onion – chopped (half of small onion)
- 1 tsp garlic powder
- 1/8 cup water
- 1/2 tsp curry powder
- 1/4 tsp cumin
- Salt/black pepper
- Preheat pan over MED heat.
- Add onion and garlic. Add 4tsp of water Cook until translucent. 5-10 min.
- Add shrimp, seasonings, and water. Mix & stir fry until cooked through.

HCG DIET RECIPE BOOK

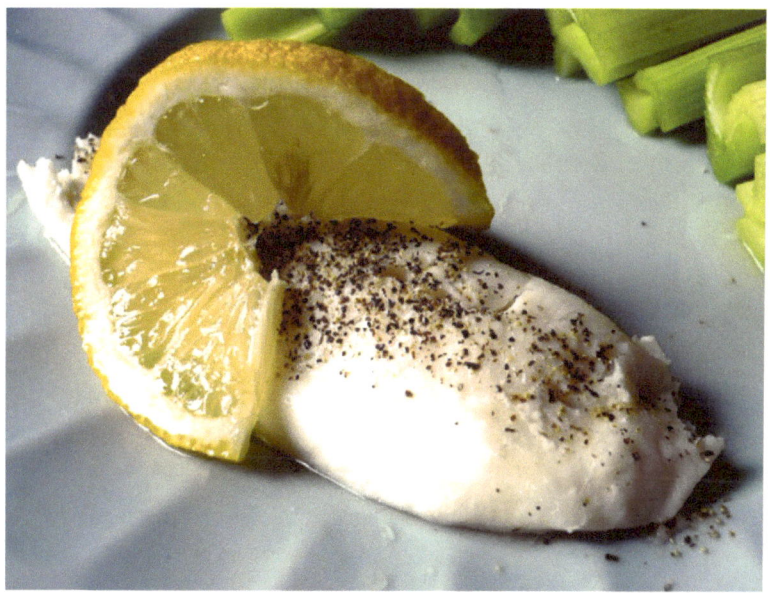

## Lemon Pepper Fish

- 100g whitefish
- Juice of half lemon
- 1 tbsp of garlic powder
- ½ tsp black pepper
- ¼ tsp salt
- ¼ tsp cumin powder

- 1/8 tsp turmeric
- Place fish in small bowl. Add garlic, black pepper, salt, cumin, and turmeric. Ensure to coat both sides.
- Cover & marinate at least 1 hour in refrigerator.
- Preheat oven to 400.
- Place the fish in a non-stick baking dish, & cover with the marinade.
- Bake 10-20 min depending on thickness, until fish easily flakes.

# NOTES

# CHAPTER TWO
# CHICKEN DISHES

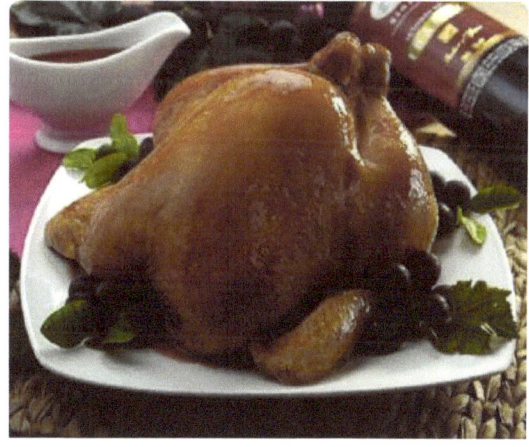

# CHINESE CHICKEN SALAD

- 100 grams of chicken chopped or shredded
- 1/3 cup chopped cabbage head
- 1/3 cup chopped lettuce head
- 1/4 cup rice vinegar
- 2 Tablespoon worsteshire souse (no fat no sugar)
- 1/4 cup Stevia

Microwave vinegar, worsteshire sauce, and STEVIA for 20-30 sec and pour over cabbage, or lettuce and chicken mixture.

Note: mixing veggies not allowed during phase 2. May use one or other.

This satisfies veggie and meat portion

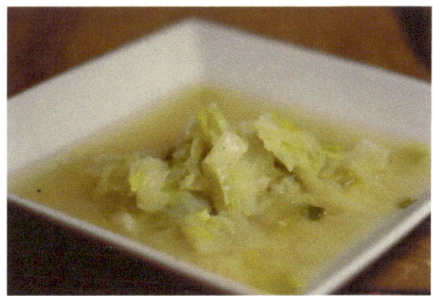

# Cabbage and Chicken Soup

- 100 g chicken
- 2 cups of chopped cabbage
- 2 cups of HCG approved chicken broth(organic free range)
- 2 cloves of minced garlic
- 1 tbsp chopped onion
- Use seasonings of choice like paprika, salt & pepper.

Heat the broth with the chicken & spices. When the chicken is cooked let it simmer for a while then add the cabbage. Cook till cabbage is tender. As the cabbage will lose some of its water & wilt there is no need to add any more water to this soup.

Notes

# Chicken con Chili

- 100g chicken
- 1 tbsp red Chile powder
- 1 tbsp ACV (apple cider vinegar)
- ½ tsp of garlic powder
- 1 tsp oregano
- 1/2 tsp cumin
- 1/2 tsp agave nectar or stevia
- Sea salt
- Crushed red pepper (optional)

In zip lock bag, add all ingredients except chicken. Mix. Sprinkle chicken with salt and add the chicken to bag. Seal & shake to coat. Place in refrigerator to marinate at least 1 hr. Cook chicken on George Foreman or under broiler until done. Top with crushed red pepper (optional) and serve.

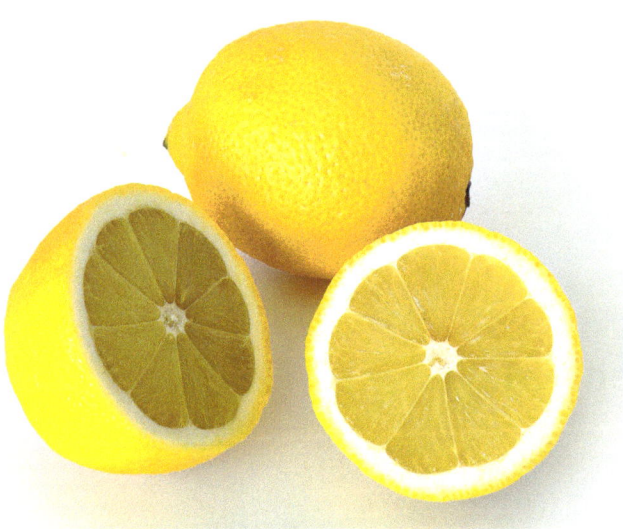

# Chicken Soup with lemon

- 100g cooked chicken breast (diced or shredded)
- Chopped spinach (allowed amount)
- 2-3 cup broth
- Juice of 1 lemon
- 1 tsp thyme
- Sea salt to taste
- Ground white pepper to taste

# Orange Ginger Chicken

- 100g chicken – cut into chunks
- Black pepper
- 1 orange – cut in ¼ parts
- 1 tsp of garlic powder
- 1 tbsp fresh ginger root (about 1/2"-1" long piece, peeled & minced)
- 1/2 tsp basil
- Juice of half lemon
- Preheat pan over MED heat.
- Sprinkle chicken with pepper.
- Add chicken to pan and stir-fry until brown on all sides, about 5-10 min.
- Add garlic powder and cook for 1 min.

- Squeeze juice of orange quarters over chicken.
- Peel & separate orange into sections. Add orange sections, ginger, lemon juice, and basil. Stir well.
- Cover and simmer for about 20-30 min.

NOTE: This includes your meat and fruit portion for this meal

# Chicken wraps

- 100 g chicken
- 2 med green cabbage leaf
- 2 med Napa cabbage leaf
- 1 tbsp of garlic powder
- 3 tbsp. balsamic vinegar
- 1 tsp onion powder
- 1 tbsp. sea salt
- 1 tbsp. pepper

Mix together garlic, onion powder, balsamic vinegar, salt, pepper and chicken pieces. Grill your chicken, and then add the Napa cabbage and cook until cabbage is slightly tender.

Take the 2 green cabbage leaves and split the chicken and spice mixture and place in cabbage leaf and roll into a wrap.

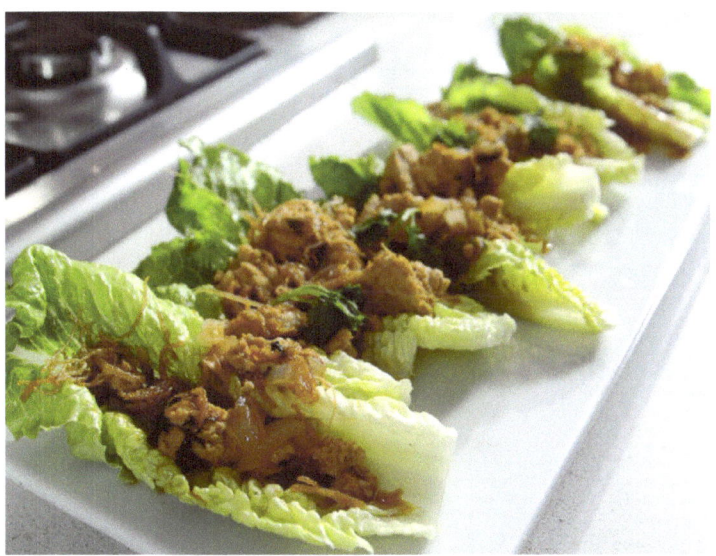

# Crunchy apple chicken salad

Ingredients

- 100 grams chicken cooked and diced
- 1 apple diced
- 3 tablespoons lemon juice
- 1/8 teaspoon cinnamon
- Dash of nutmeg
- Dash of cardamom
- Dash of salt
- Stevia to taste

- Wedge of lemon Methods/steps
- Mix ingredients together, sprinkle with stevia and cinnamon. Chill for 20 minutes.

# This page left blank for your notes

# Chapter 3
# Beef Dishes

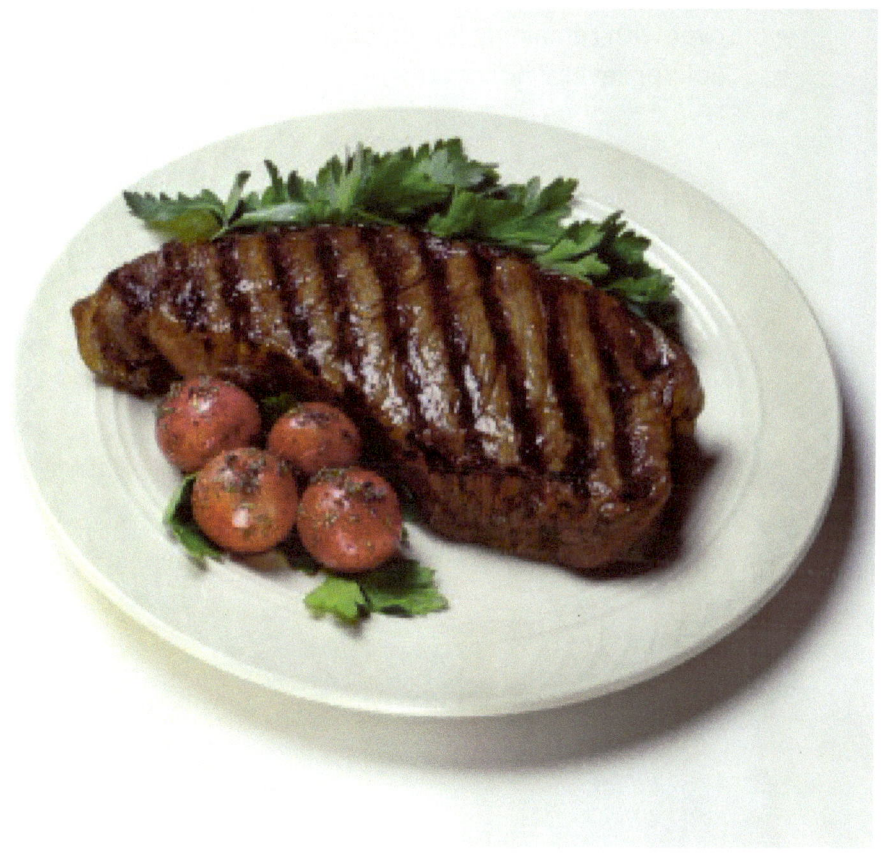

# Crock pot Roast

- 100g steak
- Onion soup mix
- 1 cup beef broth
- Black pepper to taste
- Add steak to crock-pot.
- Cover with remaining ingredients.
- Cook for several hours until reaches desired doneness.
- Serve.

.

.

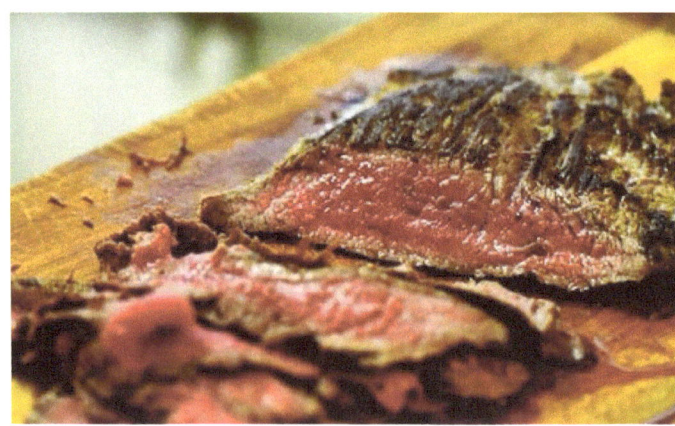

# Crock-pot Swiss steak

- 100g steak
- 1 tbsp ground melba toast
- 1 tbsp of garlic powder
- 1 stalk celery – sliced
- 1 onion – sliced
- 1 tomato – diced
- 1/2-1 cup beef broth
- Preheat pan over MED-HI heat.
- Dip steak in ground Melba toast mixture coating both sides.
- Add steak to pan and brown on both sides.
- Transfer steak to crock-pot.
- Cover with garlic, onions, or diced tomato.
- Top with beef broth (organic). Don't stir!
- Cover and cook on low until reaches desired doneness.

When done, serve immediately, and cover with juices from crock-pot

# MINI-MEAT LOAF

- 100g ground steak
- 1/2 tsp milk
- 1 grissini (ground into powder)
- 1tbsp of garlic powder
- 1/2 tsp dehydrated minced onion /or onion powder
- 1/2 tsp mustard powder
- 1/4 tsp allspice
- 1/8 tsp sage
- Salt/pepper to taste
- Any additional seasonings you like
  Preheat oven to 350.
- In small bowl, combine all ingredients and form into a small meatloaf.
- Place in glass dish, cover, and bake 25-30 mins.
- Mash up tomato and add agave nectar or stevia to make the tomato sauce.
- Uncover dish and pour sauce mix on top
- Serve immediately

NOTE: This includes your meat, grissini, vegetable and 1/2 tsp of your daily allowance of milk

# CHILI!

- 100g ground steak
- 1 tomato
- 1/2 cup water or broth
- 1 tbsp garlic powder
  Seasonings (to taste):

- 1/2 tsp onion powder
- 1/2 tsp oregano
- 1/4 tsp cumin
- 1/4 tsp black pepper
- 1/4 tsp cayenne
- 1/4 tsp basil
- 1/4 tsp thyme
- Preheat pan over MED heat.

Add garlic powder and 1 tbsp of the water/broth to pan. Stew down 2-3 mins. Add more water/broth as necessary. Increase heat to MED-HI. Add ground steak and sauté until brown – about 5 mins. Add all seasonings and cook an additional 3 mins. Continue to add more water/broth as necessary. While that is cooking dice 1/2 of tomato and place other 1/2 in food processor or blender to puree. Mix in tomatoes, puree, and rest of broth. Turn heat down to MED-LO and simmer until it reaches desired consistency.

# CABBAGE ROLLS

- 3.5 oz lean ground beef
- 1/2 Cup canned, diced tomatoes (make sure no added sugar)
- 1t Onion powder
- 1t Garlic powder
- Season salt
- Dash of Pepper
- 2 Large Cabbage leaves
- 1/2 cup chopped cabbage
- Preheat oven to 450'
- Cook beef with all spices until almost done. Add half the tomatoes and chopped cabbage cook down a bit until cabbage soft and most liquid is absorbed.
- Half the mixture and put in the two cabbage leaves.
- Wrap tucking the ends in as much as possible. (I cute the center end part of the cabbage out (the really thick part) makes it easier to wrap.
- Place 1/8 of your remaining tomatoes in small baking dish, roll around so it covers bottom, add cabbage rolls, and top with remaining 1/8 cup tomatoes.
- Bake covered for about 30 min until outer cabbage is tender.
- 2 Nice size rolls just 1 protein and 1 veggie

# CHAPTER FOUR
## QUICK MEALS

THIS CHAPTER IS FOR DAYS WHEN YOU'RE ON THE GO AND UNABLE TO COOK A MEAL. THIS I FIND IS THE WHOLE REASON WHY YOU END UP ON THE HCG DIET IN THE FIRST PLACE. YOU'RE NOT ALWAYS ABLE TO EAT WHEN YOU SHOULD AND TIME DOESN'T PERMIT IT.

# Pizza Substitute

- Prep Time:
- 5 min Cook Time:
- 10 min Ready In:
- 15 min
- Servings: 1 serving
- Ingredients
- 100 grams 97% lean ground beef
- 1 tomato (chopped to small bite size pieces)
- 1/2 sweet onion (also chopped)
- 1/2 cup homemade salsa or a red pepper (chopped)
- Salt free sugar free Italian seasoning
- Garlic powder
- Black pepper
- Cook beef, rinse, pat dry with paper towel
- Put veggies and salsa in pan and start to cook
- When the onions starts looking caramel color add beef
- Season to taste with seasonings
- Cook until most of salsa is evaporated
- Spoon onto Melba toast for a pizza like taste or eat alone, it's yummy either way!!!

Directions

Cook beef, rinse, pat dry with paper towel Put veggies and salsa in pan and start to cook When the onions starts looking caramel color add beef Season to taste with seasonings Cook until most of salsa is evaporated Spoon onto melba toast for a pizza like taste or eat alone, it's yummy either way!!!

# Not Really a Bloody Mary

- Tomato (allowed amount)
- Juice of half lemon
- 1tsp fresh cilantro, minced
- ½ tsp stevia (to taste)
- 1/4-1/2 tsp garlic paste (to taste) or 1 clove minced
- ¼ tsp cumin
- ¼ tsp sugar-free Worcestershire
- 1/8 tsp celery seed
- Salt/pepper (to taste)
- Tabasco (to taste)

In blender, combine all ingredients and puree until reaches desired consistency. Place in refrigerator until chilled or serve over ice.

TIP: Depending on the amount of tomato used, you may need to vary most of these amounts according to taste.

## Strawberry cinnamon drink

Ingredients: 10 Strawberries 2 Stevia Packets 1-2 tbsp Cinnamon Ice 1/4-1/2tsp Salt Instructions: Preparation Remove strawberry tops and discard. Wash strawberries. Cooking In a blender combine all ingredients and blend on high until a smooth consistency. Pour in a tall cup and enjoy.

# CHAPTER FIVE
## TIPS

During phase two of the HCG diet you have many questions that linger still after you leave the office of your physician. These are a few details to help you succeed with your program.

**Tip one**: everyone's experience will be different. You are unique individual follow your physicians plan for you and don't listen to others tips and etc.

**Tip two**: you cannot get HCG from the corner store. You must go to a licensed practitioner that can order pharmaceutical grade as use of anything else can gravely jeopardize your health.

**Tip three**: remember you wont be on the phase two diet forever. Sticking to the diet can help you move closer or achieve your healthcare goals so no cheating.

**Tip four**: weigh yourself daily

**Tip five**: prepare your meats and veggies every Sunday evening for the week

**Tip six**: don't do this diet without being on a medically supervised HCG program

**Tip seven**: don't eat the same meats twice a day

**Tip eight**: if you're a breakfast eater use your fruit from lunch portion for breakfast e.g.; have half of a grapefruit with agave nectar in the morning for breakfast or handful of strawberries with stevia.

**Tip nine:** eat all meals on the diet. Do not skip

**Tip ten:** have a positive outlook on what you're doing.

# CHAPTER 6
## FOOD JOURNAL

USE THESE NEXT PAGES AS YOUR DIET LOG SO
WHEN YOU RETURN FOR YOUR OFFICE VISITS YOU
CAN REVIEW WITH YOUR PRACTITIONER

| BREAKFAST | LUNCH | DINNER |
|-----------|-------|--------|
|           |       |        |
|           |       |        |

## ABOUT THE AUTHOR.

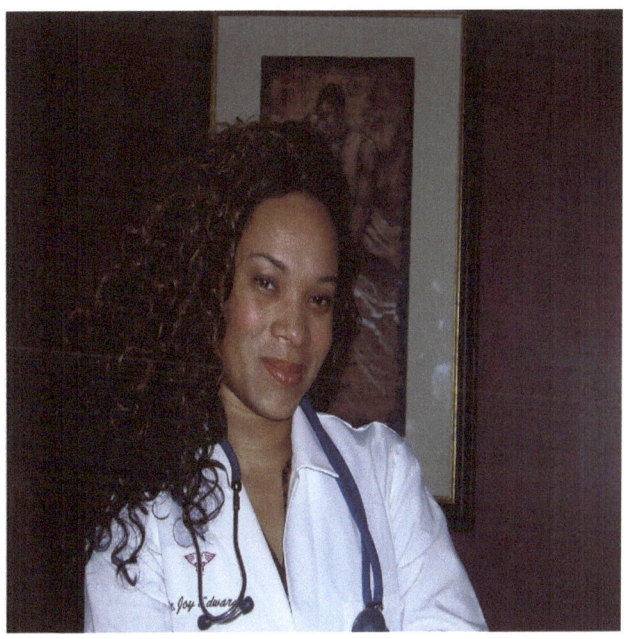

Dr. Joy Edwards NMD, HMD, MPH

Dr. Edwards journey to natural health and wellness was a truly personal experience. Diagnosed with type 2 diabetes in 2005 she suffered the depression and sadness that comes with any diagnosis of that sort. She began to gain weight and was then diagnosed with fibroids. Overweight and diabetic suffering from fibroids and extended menstrual cycles she did what anyone educated in western medicine would do, took her medication and just lived through it. It wasn't until she left her job of 5 yrs to work in plastic surgery that her life changed. This particular office was different it was a holistic cosmetics practice it had all aspects of alternative medicine combined with a surgical component. This began her journey to wellness. She began a regimen of herbs and diet changes that a yr later left her fibroid free but still overweight. At this point Dr. Joy wanted to learn more about alternative medicine. As she searched for knowledge and decided to go back to school for massage therapy, homeopathy and finally a Doctor of Natural Medicine (naturopathy). Dr. Joy then pursued a MPH to allow her to be able to conduct research using these natural treatments and helps the cause. Changing her lifestyle saved her life.

She currently has a successful alternative medicine practice in Lithia Springs and Marietta GA.

Dr. Joy completed a 1 yr residency at rejuvenation and wellness center where she worked with a MD who practiced alternative and complimentary medicine. She was trained in bio-identical hormone therapy,Chelation,plaqextherapy,Vitamintherapy.

Now Dr. Joy is free from diabetes and fibroids and no longer overweight. That's her story... Where does yours begin?

-